Abderrahim ELLAFI
Latifa MTIBAA
Boutheina JEMLI

Human myiasis

Abderrahim ELLAFI
Latifa MTIBAA
Boutheina JEMLI

Human myiasis

Four new cases in Tunisia

ScienciaScripts

Imprint

Any brand names and product names mentioned in this book are subject to trademark, brand or patent protection and are trademarks or registered trademarks of their respective holders. The use of brand names, product names, common names, trade names, product descriptions etc. even without a particular marking in this work is in no way to be construed to mean that such names may be regarded as unrestricted in respect of trademark and brand protection legislation and could thus be used by anyone.

Cover image: www.ingimage.com

This book is a translation from the original published under ISBN 978-620-6-71832-1.

Publisher:
Sciencia Scripts
is a trademark of
Dodo Books Indian Ocean Ltd. and OmniScriptum S.R.L publishing group

120 High Road, East Finchley, London, N2 9ED, United Kingdom
Str. Armeneasca 28/1, office 1, Chisinau MD-2012, Republic of Moldova, Europe
Printed at: see last page
ISBN: 978-620-8-24688-4

TABLE OF CONTENTS

INTRODUCTION

Myiasis is a cosmopolitan ectoparasitosis caused by acephalous and apodous larvae (maggots) of cyclorrhagic diptera (flies). [1].

Recognized since ancient times, the flies responsible for myiasis are among the world's most devastating insects, causing severe losses in animal husbandry, with major economic losses ,including reduced milk production, weight problems, fertility and poor leather quality [1].

In mammals (including humans), Dipteran larvae can feed on the dead tissue, liquid body substances or ingested food of the host and can cause a wide range of infestations, depending on the location of the body and the relationship of the larvae to the host [2]. Human myiasis is mainly caused by flies belonging to the *Calliphoridae, Oestridae or* Sarcophaginae families [3]. The distribution of human myiasis is worldwide, with more species and greater abundance in the poorer socio-economic regions of tropical and subtropical countries.

Infestation is not necessarily linked to the tropical world, but travel to one of these destinations may increase the risk of myiasis, particularly cutaneous myiasis. [4]. In countries where it is not endemic, myiasis is an important condition, and may represent the fourth most common skin disease associated with travel [[5].

Travel has clearly highlighted the importance of myiasis awareness, particularly in countries where infestation is unusual and rare.

Even physicians unfamiliar with this disease can easily diagnose cases in which mygots are visible, but furuncular, migratory and cavitary cases and pseudomyiasis pose a diagnostic challenge. Clinicians need to be aware of the possibility of this diagnosis, as timely and appropriate treatment can reduce lesion extension and morbidity [6]. For a correct diagnosis, several aspects need to be determined: the region the patient has visited, the climatic conditions and the habits of the species in the region visited. An accurate and rapid diagnosis is important not only to alleviate the patient's symptoms, but also to prevent the prescription of unnecessary treatments, particularly antibiotics, which encourage the development of bacterial resistance. Increased world trade, immigration and global warming will also increase the likelihood of myiasis-causing flies spreading to new territories, or to regions where they were already eradicated in the past - hence the important role of physicians in active surveillance. [7].

The aim of our work was to study the epidemiological, clinical and biological characteristics of myiasis, as well as its treatment, by reporting four cases of myiasis diagnosed in the parasitology-mycology laboratory of the main military training hospital in Tunis.

METHODS

Type of study:

This was a retrospective and descriptive study. It involved four cases of myiasis diagnosed at the Parasitology-Mycology Laboratory of the Tunis Main Military Training Hospital between 2018 and 2022.

1. Study population:

We included all clinically suspected cases of human myiasis with parasitological confirmation at the Tunis Military Hospital during the study period. Species diagnosis was based on macroscopic and microscopic criteria according to Zumpt's criteria.

Observations were completed with all the patient's clinical information, management and evolution.

2. Data collection:

For each case, we recorded sex, age, country of residence, pathological history, clinical signs, myiasis species, any complications, treatment modalities and clinical course.

3. Bibliographic research:

We used the electronic databases PubMed, Science direct and Google Scholar, to select articles of interest. The keywords used were: human myiasis, travel, Tunisia, as well as their corollaries in English. We also consulted the register of theses and dissertations of the four faculties of medicine.

4. Ethical considerations and declaration of interests:

As this was a retrospective study, the consent of the patients reported was not sought. However, anonymity and confidentiality of personal data were respected.

RESULTS

1. Comments:

1.1. Comment 1:

This was a 38-year-old female patient, a worker at Djerba airport, followed up for bilateral tympanic perforation following recurrent otitis and antisynthetase syndrome evolving for 5 years under corticosteroid and immunosuppressive treatment.

In June 2018, while hospitalized for her monthly course of Cyclophosphamide, the patient presented with clear rhinorrhea with nocturnally exacerbating nasal pruritus. There was no fever or other clinical signs. Two days after the onset of rhinorrhea, the patient noticed the presence of mobile, whitish worms measuring a few millimeters in length when blowing her nose. The ENT examination showed only an appearance consistent with congestive rhinitis, with no other abnormalities. Biological workup was without abnormalities, notably no hypereosinophilia or inflammatory syndrome.

Macroscopic and microscopic examination of 2 larvae enabled them to be identified according to Zumpt's criteria. These were L2 stage larvae (5 and 6 mm) of *Oestrus ovis* **(figure 1).** The larvae are semi-cylindrical in shape. The pseudocephalon has two buccal hooks **(figure 2).** The posterior respiratory stigmas are subcircular with a central knob, pierced by numerous pores **(figure 3). The diagnosis of nasal myiasis was retained.**

The patient received saline as a nasal lavage several times a day. The evolution was favorable, with no recurrence. The follow-up was 3 years.

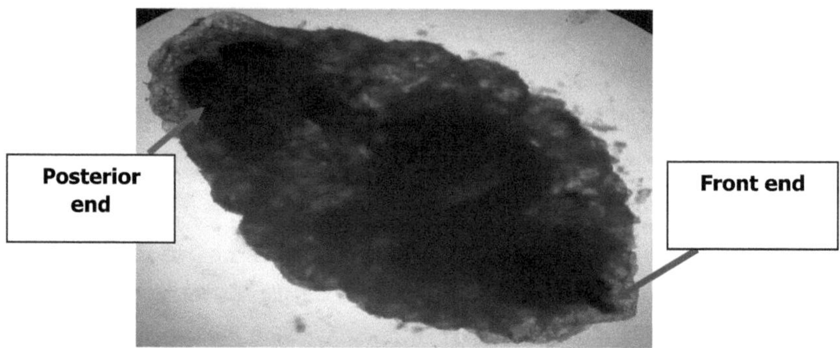

Figure 1: *Oestrus ovis* larva stage L2 [6mm] [photo taken at the HMPIT parasitology laboratory].

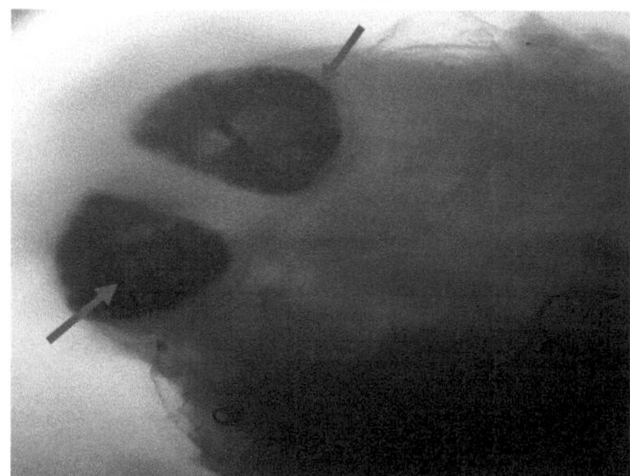

Figure 2: Posterior end of larva: respiratory stigmata [red arrows] [photo taken at the HMPIT parasitology laboratory].

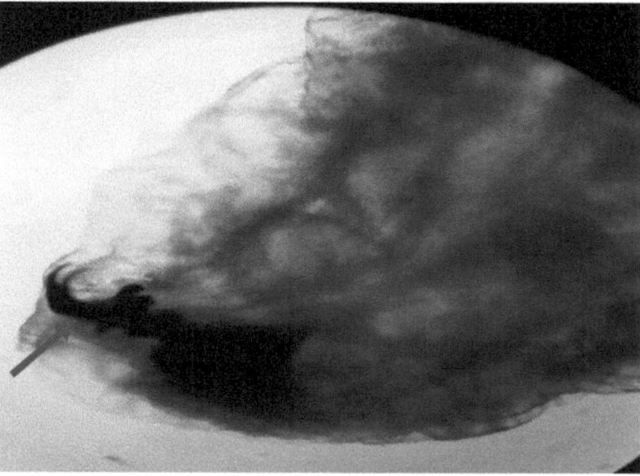

Figure 3: Anterior end of larva: mouth hooks [blue arrow] [photo taken at the HMPIT parasitology laboratory].

1.2. Comment 2:

The patient was 50 years old, a worker at Tunis airport, with no notable pathological history.

She presented with a 10-day history of influenza-like illness with polyarthralgia, coughing fits and purulent sputum, in a context of apyrexia. The patient also noticed the emission of millimetric, whitish-colored worms when coughing. This prompted her to seek medical advice.

ENT examination showed only pharyngitis with congestive mucosa on nasal endoscopy. Pulmonary auscultation was unremarkable, with a normal chest X-ray. Biology was unremarkable, with no hypereosinophilia or biological inflammatory syndrome. Chest X-ray was normal.

Parasitological examination identified L2 [8mm] stage *Oestrus ovis* larvae **(figure 4)**. The larvae were semi-cylindrical in shape. The diagnosis of nasopharyngeal myiasis was accepted.

The patient was given an antiseptic mouthwash and saline solution as a nasal wash several times a day. The evolution was favorable after 15 days, with no new worms emitted.

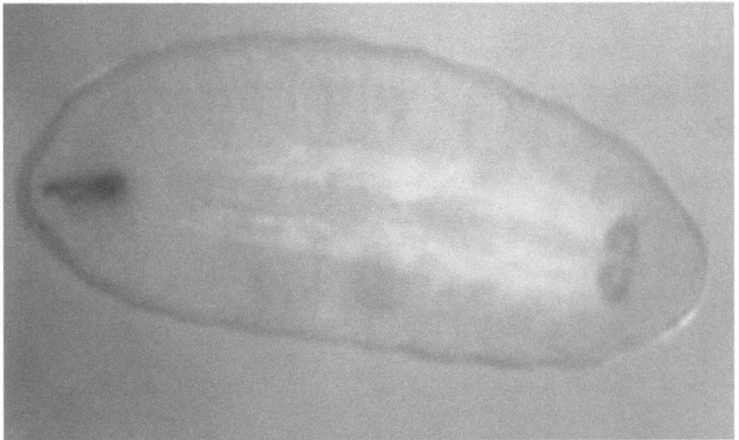

Figure 4: *Oestrus ovis* larva L2 stage [8 mm] (photo taken at the HMPIT parasitology laboratory)

1.3. Comment 3 [[8]:

The patient was 60 years old, male, from Bizerte. His history included type 2 diabetes for 28 years, at the stage of degenerative complications; arterial hypertension for 4 years; coronary artery disease and chronic renal failure for two years.

He was admitted to the Infectious Diseases Department of the Tunis Military Hospital in September 2019 for management of a diabetic foot wound. He underwent amputation of the second, third and fourth toes of his right foot. After two months, he began hyperbaric oxygen therapy (HBOT) sessions, during which a mobile whitish worm was observed in the wound **(figure 5).**

The laboratory work-up showed no abnormalities, notably no hypereosinophilia or biological inflammatory syndrome.

The larvae were collected and transferred to the parasitology department. Species identification was carried out according to Zumpt's criteria. The larvae were stage L3 *Lucilia sericata* **(figure 5).**

The larva was 12 mm long. Its shape was semi-cylindrical with a tapering anterior end containing buccal hooks **(Figure 6).** At the posterior end of the larva were the respiratory stigmata. These posterior spiracles contained a narrow peritreme that formed a fully enclosed ring, also surrounding a conspicuous knob **(figure 7).**

In addition to mechanical removal of the larvae using clinical forceps, the lesion was rinsed with an aqueous chlorhexidine solution® and no systemic treatment was administered.

The dressing was changed twice a day. No larval infestation was observed during evolution. Wound healing was accelerated by HBOT, with a good clinical outcome.

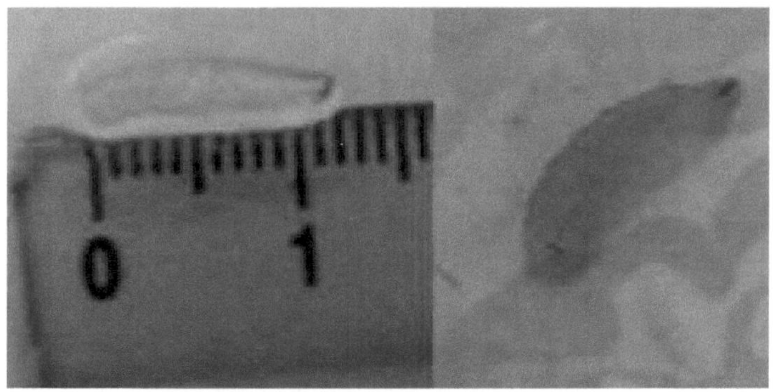

Figure 5: *Lucilia Sericata* L3 stage larva

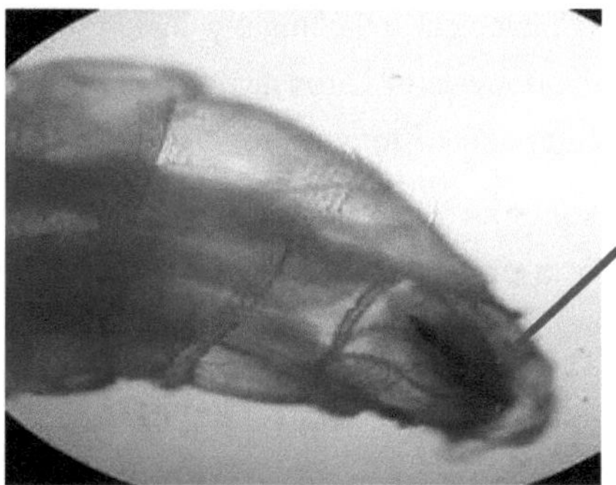

Figure 6: Cephalic end of the *Lucilia sericata* larva: mouth hooks [blue arrow].

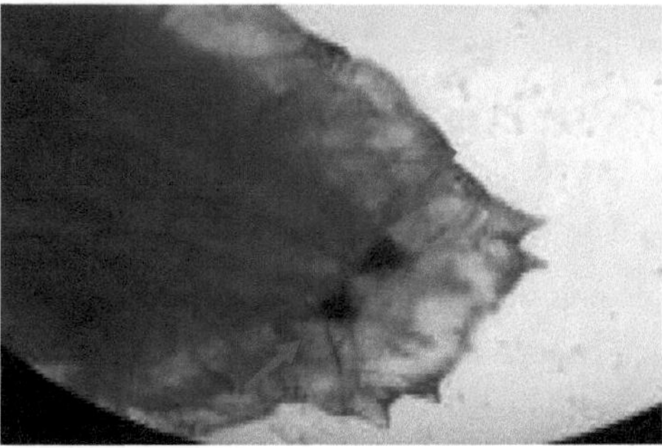

Figure 7: Posterior end of *Lucilia sericata* larva: respiratory stigmata (red arrows)

(Photos taken at the HMPIT parasitology laboratory)

1.4. **Comment 4** [[9]:

The patient is 31 years old, with no previous pathological history. He was the victim of a road accident (collision between two cars) on November 02, 2021.

The patient was referred to the nearest emergency department with admission examination: Glasgow score 4/15, pupils in tight miosis, Polypnea at 22 cycles per minute, SpO2 88% on room air, bilateral snoring rales and tachycardia. The patient was intubated. He had a bodyscan which showed a meningeal hemorrhage and fractures to the cervical vertebrae C5/C6. The patient remained in the emergency department for 36 hours before being admitted to the intensive care unit of the Tunis Military Hospital (Day 0). On the second day, the evolution was marked by the onset of fever (39.8°C) and a biological inflammatory syndrome with hyperleukocytosis (16200 cells/mm3) and high levels of C-reactive protein (360mg/l) and procalcitonin (34 µg/l). He was put on augmentin® for suspected aspiration pneumonitis.

An infectious investigation was ordered, including microbiological examination of cerebrospinal fluid, urine, a protected tracheal specimen and blood culture. On the third day, due to persistent septic shock, the patient was started on Tazocillin and Vancomycin.

On the same day and after the patient had been cared for (shower, diaper change, etc.), the nurse reported the presence of a multitude of small, sticky white worms in the patient's intimate areas (anal margin), which were collected and sent to the parasitology laboratory for identification.

Biological analyses showed a biological inflammatory syndrome with hyperleukocytosis (16,200 cells/mm3) and high levels of C-reactive protein (360mg/l) and procalcitonin (34 µg/l).

According to Zumpt's criteria, the larval specimens were identified as *Musca domestica* larval stage L3 (8 mm) **(figure 8).** The anterior end of the larva was tapered and contained a pair of hooks **(figure 9).** The posterior end was broad and flattened with spiracles that have three sinuous slits surrounded by a heavily sclerotized ring with a conspicuous perforated knob **(Figure 10).**

Intimate areas were shaved with conventional cleansing and antiseptic disinfection. The patient's condition worsened dramatically and he died on the 4th day from septic shock and multiple visceral failures.

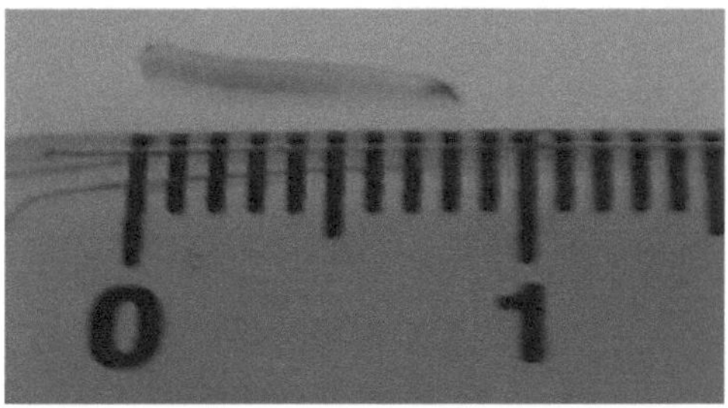

Figure 8: *Musca domestica* L3 stage larva [8mm].

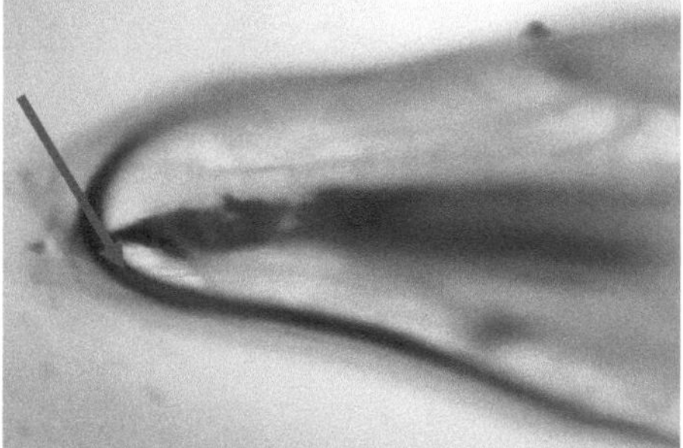

Figure 9: Tapering anterior end of the *Musca domestica* larva containing a pair of hooks [blue arrow].

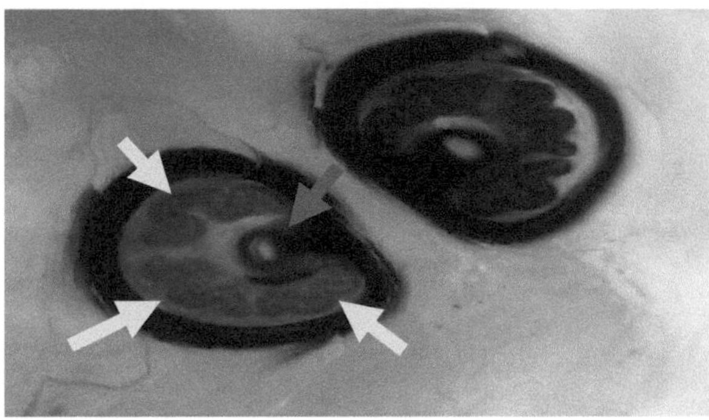

Figure 10: The posterior end of the *Musca domestica* larva shows: a pair of brown 'D'-shaped respiratory spiracles, a chitinized ring (red arrow) and 3 sinuous 'm'-shaped stigmatic slits on each spiracle (yellow arrows).

(Photos taken at the HMPIT parasitology laboratory)

DISCUSSION

Human myiasis is a disease rarely seen in Tunisia. In this paper, we report four cases of human myiasis diagnosed in Tunisians at the Tunis Military Hospital. The average age of these patients was 45, with a sex ratio of 1. No notion of travel was reported in our patients, but two of our patients worked at the airport. Both had **Oestrus ovis** nasal myiasis. The third patient had **Lucilia sericata** myiasis in a diabetic foot sore. Finally, we report the first Tunisian case of nosocomial **Musca domestica** myiasis found in the private parts of a patient hospitalized in intensive care.

As flies are distributed throughout the world, myiasis is cosmopolitan. Maggots can remain on the surface of the skin (epicutaneous hematophagous myiasis: case worm), dig up jokes (*Lucilia spp.* larvotherapy), penetrate cavities (*Oestrus ovis* in the nose or eye), penetrate the skin (subcutaneous myiasis, either furunculous, Cayor worm or macaque worm, or crawling: *Gasterophilus*),or perform an internal tissue cycle (*Hypoderma* in parasitic deadlock in humans) [10].

The classic fly cycle **(figure 11):** after mating, females lay their eggs on the substrate most suitable for their offspring (soil, often putrid water, stems, flower buds, fruit or vegetables, etc.), either singly, in streaks or scattered over a larger or smaller surface area. After a variable length of time, from a few minutes to over six months, the egg hatches, giving rise to a larva (maggot), measuring from a few millimeters to around 2 cm. At the posterior end of the larva is a pair of respiratory stigmata, the morphology of which varies according to genus and species. After a period of time, often depending on ambient temperature, and a number of moults that allow the maggot to reach full development, its cuticle hardens: this is the pupa. Inside the pupa, the adult insect (or imago) forms. At maturity, the fly escapes through a preformed operculum, and the cycle begins anew. [10,11].

Male flies are generally smaller and emerge earlier than females. As a general rule, with an adequate larval diet, the parasite spends more time in the nymph stage than in the egg or larva stage. Adult longevity varies according to environmental conditions.

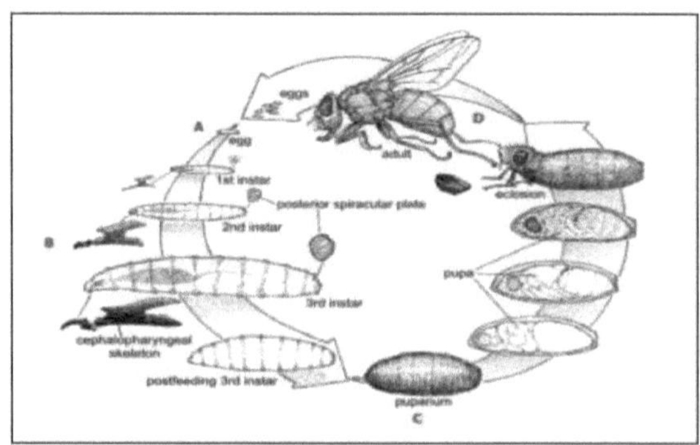

Figure 11: Life cycle of myiasis flies A: egg, B: larva [3 stages], C: pupa, D: adult [12].

Human myiasis is classified according to the type of parasitism involved:

- **Compulsory myiasis** responsible for furunculosis in the tropics (*Dermatobia hominis, Cordylobia anthropophaga*) and visceral forms (*Hypoderma bovis*).

- **Accidental** or **opportunistic human myiasis** affects natural cavities: auricular, rhino-ocular (*Oestrus ovis, Rhinoestrus purpureus*), genital (*Musca domestica*), rectal (*Eristalis tenax*), skin folds and wounds (*Lucilia, Calliphora, Wohlfahrtia, Cochlyomyia*). [13].

The clinical manifestations of myiasis vary according to the species of fly, the number of larvae and the location of the invaded area [14]. **Table I** summarizes the main human myiasis cases according to the clinical entity, type of parasitism, geographical distribution and species involved.

Table 1: Main myiasis diseases encountered in human pathology [10]:

Clinical entities	Type of parasitism	Species or genus	Geographical distribution
Hematophagous epicutans	Mandatory	*Auchmeromyia senegalensis*	Black Africa
Folds	Opportunistic	*Musca domestica* *Calliphora erythrocephala*	Cosmopolitan
Wounds	Opportunistic Mandatory	*Musca* spp. and *Calliphora* spp, *Lucilia* spp. *Cochliomyia hominivorax*	Cosmopolitan America
Fungus	Mandatory	*Hypoderma bovis* *Cordylobia anthropophaga* *Dermatobia hominis*	Black Africa Europe Latin America
Conjunctival	Mandatory	*OEstrus ovis*	Mediterranean basin
Creeping subcutaneous	Mandatory	*Gasterophilus intestinalis*	Cosmopolitan
Cavity: -vagina -rectum -ear canal -Sinus, nose	Opportunistic Opportunistic Opportunistic Mandatory	*Musca domestica* *Eristalis tenax* *Musca* spp, *Calliphora* spp, *Lucilia* spp. *OEstrus ovis,* *Rhinoestrus*	Cosmopolitan Europe Cosmopolitan Europe[south],Africa
Intraocular	Mandatory	*Hypoderma bovis*	Europe
Central nervous system	Mandatory	*Hypoderma bovis*	Europe

The clinical diagnosis of "myiasis" is obvious if one or more maggots are visible at the bottom of an opening, or are brought in by the patient.

In **hypodermosis**, major blood and/or meningeal hyper-eosinophilia may point to a diagnosis, but the diagnosis of certainty is based on serology and rarely on larval identification. In the event of a positive result, regular fundus monitoring should be instituted.

Gasterophilus **creeping myiasis** should be suspected when a patient caring for horses or living in the countryside near an equine breeding station has a migratory groove in the neck or upper thorax and has not travelled to a tropical zone (elimination of a larbish (hookworm) and a larva currens (anguillula).

In other myiasis cases, the diagnosis is made by visualizing the maggots. These are removed with forceps or a blunt curette **(figure 12)** (conjunctival myiasis, wounds, skin folds, natural cavities, etc.), or after excision in the case of furunculous myiasis, or by expulsion during sneezing or nose blowing in the case of nasal and sinus myiasis, or in the stool in the case of digestive or rectal myiasis (*Erystalis tenax, Fannia* spp). The latter can sometimes be seen during rectoscopy or low colonoscopy and extirpated during examination[13].

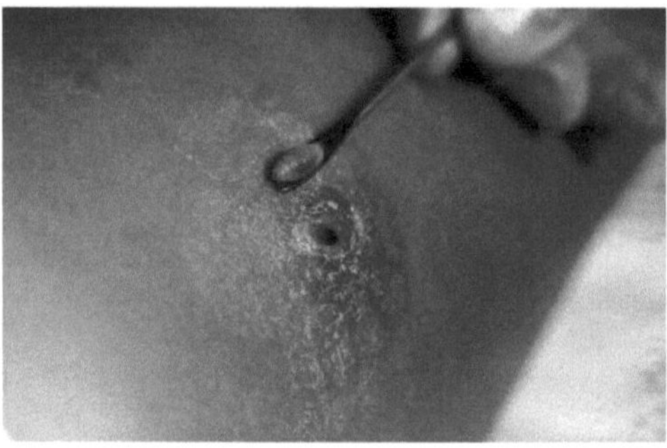

Figure 12: *Cordylobia anthropophaga* larva extracted on a foam curette[13]

For entomological diagnosis, collected maggots must be fixed with 70° ethyl alcohol. Except in special cases, identification of the species in question requires the help of an experienced entomologist. Identification is carried out on stage III larvae (except for *Hypoderma bovis*, which is stage I). Size, shape, color and ornamentation all play a part in identification. But it's essentially by observing the posterior end where the respiratory stigmas (or spiracles) are located, whose morphology varies according to genus and species, that identification can be made with certainty. A spiracle consists of a sclerotized peritreme and circular structure or "button" surrounding (except in *Oestridae* and *Hypodermatidae*) the respiratory slits (one in stage I, two in stage II and three in stage III, the most characteristic stage) **(Figure 13).** Identification is also based on the shape of the buccal sclerites (hooks) at the anterior end. After dissection and dehydration, identification involves mounting the ends of the larvae between slide and coverslip, in Canada Balsam [10]. An identification key based on clinical forms is given in **Appendix 1**.

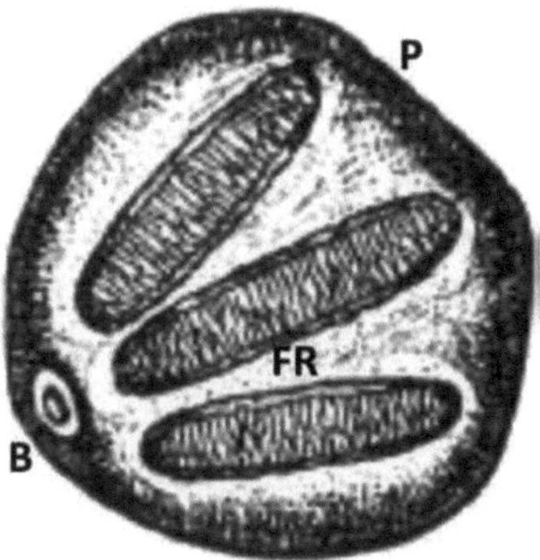

Figure 13: Classic morphology of respiratory stigmata in cyclorrhoea flies. P: peritreme; B: button; FR: respiratory slits (or stigmata)[[10].

In this dissertation, we report the first cases of ***Oestrus ovis*** nasal myiasis in Tunisia.

Oestrus ovis is the most isolated species in myiasis, and is responsible for a generally benign infection. It belongs to the *Oestridae* family, subfamily *Oestrinae*. It is an almost cosmopolitan dipteran insect. It is distributed throughout the subtropics. The majority of cases reported in the literature come from North Africa, South Asia and the Middle East. [15]. With its atrophied mouthparts, this small greyish-yellow fly does not feed and leads a very short life, devoted solely to reproduction. [16] **(figure 14).**

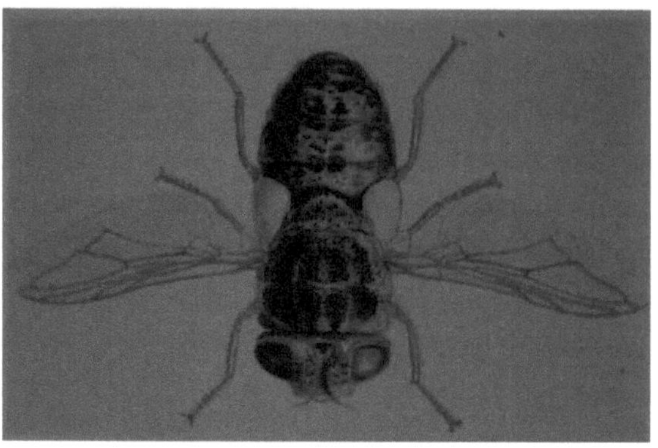

Figure 14: The *Oestrus* Ovis fly [17].

The larvae of these flies, obligatory parasites of sheep, travel up to the frontal sinuses to continue their development. Their passage through the nasal cavities of sheep and goats causes agitation and sneezing. Their presence in the sinuses causes dizziness and stimulates mucus secretion in both animals and humans. In their final stage of development, the larvae are shed into the nasal mucus (jetage disease). L1 larvae, deposited in September-October, undergo hypobiosis for two to 12 months and are released into the nasal mucus the following spring. They fall to the ground, where they pupate. Pupation is dependent on favorable climatic conditions and lasts from 30 to 35 days; in July-August, the pupa gives rise to an adult insect or imago[16] **(figures 14, 15 and 16).**

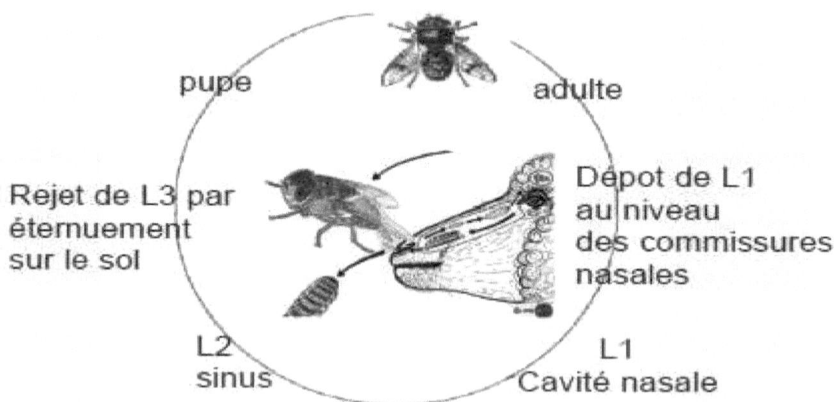

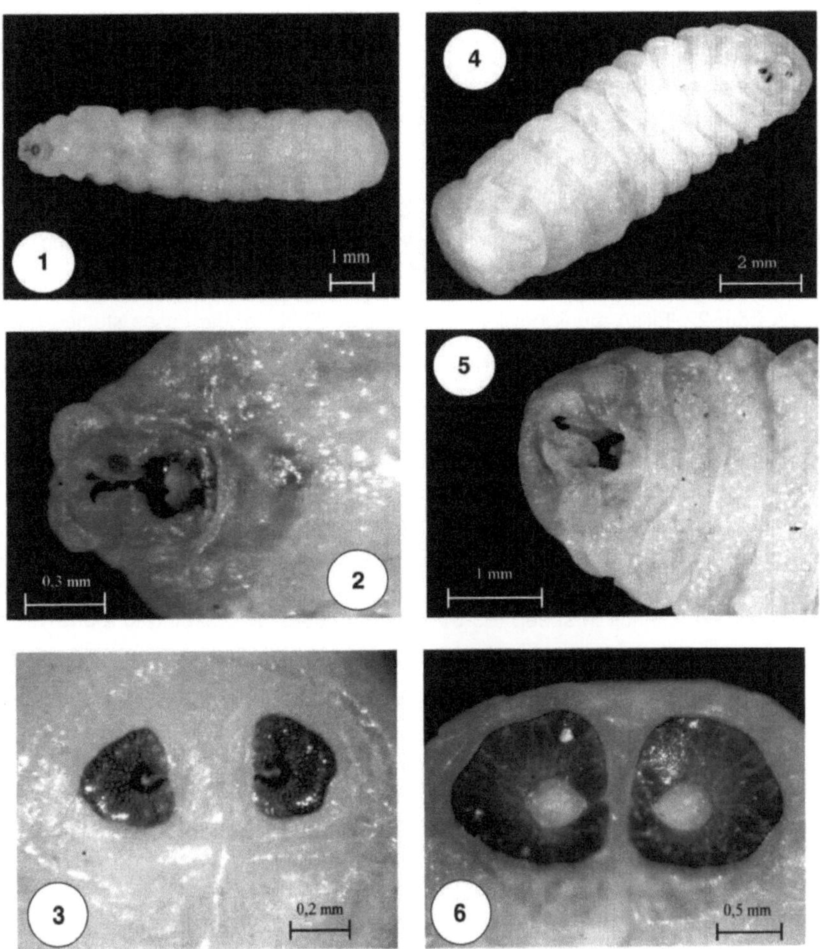

Figure 16: *Oestrus* ovis larvae *[16]*.

Images 1-3: Second larval stage or L2.

Image 1: Ventral view; Image 2: Buccal hooks; Image 3: Posterior peritremes.

Images 4-6: Third larval stage or L3.

Image 4: Ventral view; Image 5: Buccal hooks; Image 6: Posterior peritremes.

The actual number of cases, both worldwide and in Tunisia, is certainly higher than the number of published cases. In Tunisia, these diseases are not notifiable. As a result, their actual prevalence among Tunisian travellers or subjects from endemic areas may be underestimated, explaining the very low number of cases reported. These low prevalences may also be explained by ignorance of the diagnosis or by extirpation of the parasites, without entomological confirmation of the diagnosis. Hence the difficulty of assessing the frequency of this condition. Classically, there is a risk factor linked to certain professions (shepherds or veterinarians in particular) and certain lifestyles, such as camping and travel to endemic areas. A study carried out by Pampiglione et al. on 112 shepherds from 22 Italian municipalities reported that 80.3% of the cases studied had contracted an *O. ovis* infection at least once in their lives. [19]. However, O. ovis can be contracted in places where there is a total absence of sheep, such as towns and beaches.

The frequency of this condition in humans is greater "where sheep are scarce and the population dense." [20]. Pagès also echoed Sergent's hypothesis, saying that "estrosis attacks man only where sheep are scarce", i.e., where the sheep population is much less dense than the human population. [21].

Despite a high prevalence in sheep (93.63%) in our country, according to a one-year study by Kilani et al, few human cases have been described. Anane and Ben Hssine reported 11 cases of conjunctival myiasis in southern Tunisia in 2010, and Zayani et al reported 23 cases in 1989 in the Tunisian Sahel, all due to *O. ovis* [22-24].

Our first two cases involved employees at the airports on the island of Djerba and Tunis Carthage, which are not sheep-breeding areas. This reinforces the hypothesis that these two cases were probably due to travel.

In humans, the cycle is always abortifacient and the larva does not go beyond stage 1 or even stage 2, as in our first two patients, but there are a few rare cases reported in the literature where *O. ovis* larvae at nasal level have been extracted at stage L3 [10,16,25-27].

In nasal myiasis, maggots cause extensive necrosis, desquamation and destruction of intranasal tissues, and can reach deep, inaccessible areas of the nose and paranasal sinuses. It has been observed that in the case of human myiasis, the majority of deaths result from involvement of the nasal cavities, with a fatality rate of up to 1.19% [28,29]. There are reports of cases of nasal myiasis extending to the oesophagus and even the stomach, with fatal outcomes resulting from tissue destruction [30]. Other complications may arise, such as infections of the orbit or facial cellulitis, ulceration of the posterior pharyngeal wall, perforation of the nasal septum, palatal perforation and, in extreme cases, penetration of the central nervous system, meningitis or pneumocephalus [29,31,32]. However, most cases are detected early due to intense discomfort, and treated before other deeper structures are affected.

Agents reported to cause nasal myiasis *include Oestrus ovis, Cochliomyia. hominivorax, Chrysomya bezziana, Lucilia sericata, Drosophila melanogaster,* and *Calliphora vicina.*

Treatment relies mainly on manual extraction of all larvae, even in deep-seated areas, which makes this method very difficult without endoscopic assistance, sometimes requiring several sessions.

Furthermore, a 2018 Indian study evaluating the efficacy of ivermectin versus manual larval extraction found that per os ivermectin was effective in the treatment of nasal and nasopharyngeal myiasis, in terms of early elimination, reduced morbidity and shorter hospital stay [33].

Curative and preventive treatment of herds with ivermectin (200 µg/kg) seems to effectively reduce infestation for all three larval stages [[34,35]. This treatment could have an impact on the frequency of human estrosis, by at least reducing the risk of contamination from cattle.

Our third case was a **Lucilia sericata** myiasis on a diabetic foot. *Lucilia* is a genus of Diptera *in the Calliphoridae* family **(figure 17).** It is a relatively small, homogeneous group of flies with a beautiful metallic blue-green color. They are, along with other genera, commonly referred to as "Green Flies" and have a predominantly saprophagous and necrophagous behavior [36].

Lucilia spp. eggs are laid on the host. Adult flies are highly sensitive to chemical stimuli and are able to easily locate suitable oviposition sites [37]. Wounds with necrotic areas are ideal sites for egg deposition and larval development **(figure 18).** The speed of development after oviposition depends on temperature. Above 30°C, incubation of *L. sericata* eggs took 10-12 hours and completion of the larval feeding stage an additional two to five days [[38]giving a total of three days for the end of feeding. Greenberg [[39] reported that the average minimum time from egg laying to completion of the second larval instar was just over two days (50 hours) at 29°C.

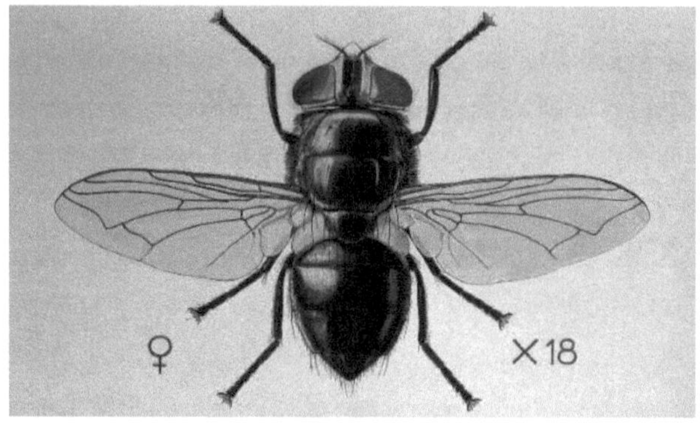

Figure 17: The Lucilia sericata fly [40]

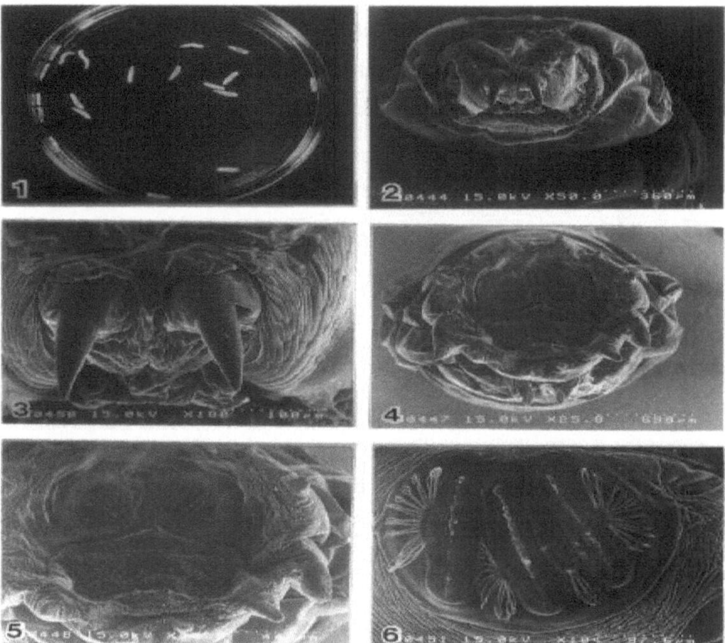

Figure 18: Lucilia sericata larvae: Images 2-6 Scanning electron microscopy of larva; 2 Anterior end with oral hooks [×50]; 3 Oral hooks [×180]; 4 Caudal end with posterior spiracles. Spiracular area surrounded by 10 tubercles [×25]; 5. Posterior spiracles with three slit-shaped openings [×50]; 6. Posterior spiracles [×180].*[41]*

Interestingly, *L. sericata* is most often used therapeutically for a variety of indications, including the treatment of osteomyelitis wounds [13]. There are three main beneficial effects of maggot therapy on a wound: debridement of necrotic tissue, disinfection by bacterial digestion, and improved wound healing by stimulating granulation tissue growth [14].

In addition, knowledge of the life cycle of *L. sericata* can improve forensic research in rural and urban areas. Sequence data of *L. sericata* as a specific marker for identification, seems to provide a valuable investigative tool in forensic entomology[42]. Insect multiplication is linked to time of death.

Traumatic or wound myiasis involves the infestation of traumatic lesions by parasitic Diptera larvae. The infestation of neglected human wounds by fly larvae during periods of war was a commonly observed phenomenon [[43] however, infestation of infected wounds by maggots in normal times is not uncommon. The smallest wound or abrasion, even that caused by a tick bite, can be a sufficient site of attraction for oviposition by the female fly. Neglected open wounds are one of the predisposing factors for myiasis. In developing countries such as India, myiasis is a sign of neglected wound care [43]. Patients were often of low socio-economic status, homeless or drug addicts. Eggs are laid in or near the wound, and the developing larvae cause severe damage through their feeding activity. The earliest case of human traumatic myiasis due to *Lucilia cuprina* was reported in West Africa in a patient suffering from leprosy [44].

Because of peripheral neuropathy, diabetic cases are considered a major risk group for the disease due to decreased sensitivity [42] as is the case for our patient.

A study by Usyal et al of 18 cases of myiasis in patients with diabetic feet found that this disease is frequently associated with poor hygiene conditions and is more common in summer. [42].

Open wounds or skin alterations not only increase the risk of human myiasis; flies' first contact with a wound can also theoretically lead to infections with antimicrobial-resistant bacteria [45-47]. A review by Onwugamba et al in 2018 showed that extended-spectrum beta-lactamase [ESBL]-producing *Escherichia coli* resistant to carbapenems or colistin, ESBL-producing *Enterococcus faecium*, *Klebsiella pneumoniae*, *Salmonella enterica* or methicillin-resistant *Staphylococcus aureus* could be detected in and on flies [48]. Although direct transmission of these bacteria between flies and humans has yet to be proven as a disease trigger, flies are at least responsible for the transmission of *Chlamydia trachomatis*, which causes trachoma [49-51]. It is therefore conceivable that, in addition to myiasis, other infections can also be transmitted by flies.

The recommended treatment in these cases of myiasis is to collect all visible larvae directly from the wound and perform active debridement and daily dressing with cleansing with antiseptic solutions; if possible, the infested area should be completely removed [52,53]. Excisions can also be made to reach the larvae. First, the larvae are forced to the surface by inducing regional hypoxia with a toxic substance; then, the larvae on the surface are cleaned mechanically [14].

It may be necessary to aerate the wound site to avoid complications such as maceration. If the wound is left open for aeration, it should be covered with a thin layer of sterile gauze. The pores of the gauze should be small enough to prevent flies from entering, while still allowing air to circulate. In addition, chronic wounds should be treated at least once a day, and closed tightly. The wound site must be inspected and cleaned regularly, to prevent the occurrence of myiasis. [42].

Our fourth case was a nosocomial **Musca domestica** myiasis of the private parts of an ICU patient.

The housefly, *Musca domestica Linnaeus* **(figure 19)**, is a cosmopolitan synanthropic species that lives in close contact with man. It is generally regarded as a mechanical vector of disease, and is capable of transferring hundreds of pathogenic organisms to humans. *Musca domestica* is also attracted to human food sources or animal waste [54,55]. The housefly, as an opportunistic species, can lay its eggs in various types of moist and decaying organic matter, such as compost, garbage, excrement, fresh and decaying fruit, most human foods and even carrion. In some cases, it can cause myiasis. The localizations reported in the literature were: intestinal, wound and cavitary [14].

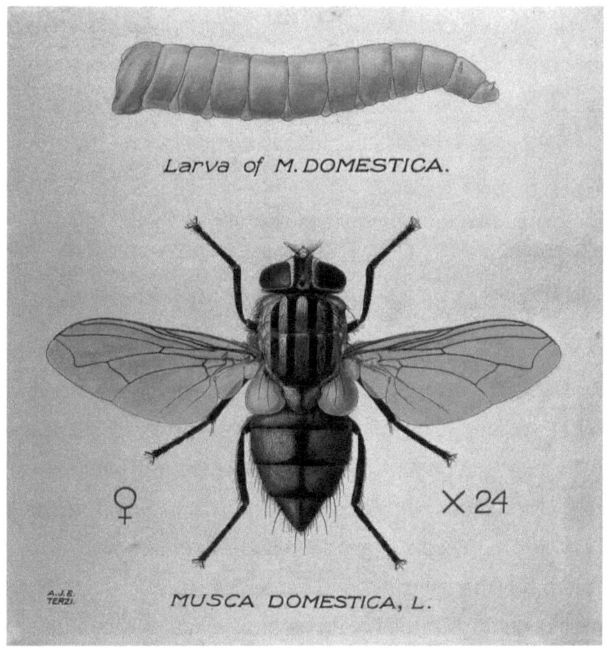

Figure 19: The larva and the *Musca* domestica fly [56].

Nosocomial myiasis or healthcare-associated myiasis is a rare entity, with only a few cases published in the literature. It can have a major psychological impact on patients and their families, and can seriously damage the hospital's image and reputation. The hospital's license and financial situation are also at stake. The factors contributing most to nosocomial myiasis are as follows. [[57]:

(i)   An altered state of consciousness or reduced mobility.

(ii)   The presence of exposed wounds or necrotic tissue.

(iii)   Poor hygiene standards.

(iv)   No barred windows.

(v)   Warm climate.

In the majority of cases of nosocomial myiasis in Europe, the most important factors were the absence of barred windows, the presence of an infected ulcer, and the absence of air conditioning in the hospital (windows had to remain open in hot weather). [58]. In developing countries, the most important factors were open windows and poor hygiene conditions [59]. In the presence of these contributing factors, myiasis can be considered a risk for patients suffering from trauma and reduced mobility. Five cases of nosocomial myiasis related to diabetic complications (two foot wounds, one leg, one nose and one eyelid) were reported by Joo and Kim [41] thus supporting the inclusion of diabetic patients among those at risk of myiasis.

To avoid myiasis, Sherman et al. [57] recommended that wounds should never be left uncovered. However, M. Dutto previously described a case of myiasis due to *Sarcophaga cruentata* in a covered wound in a polytrauma patient hospitalized in the intensive care unit [60]. The same author, accompanied by M. Pellegrino and S. Vanin, decided to carry out a simple experiment to confirm the ability of first-stage *Sarcophaga* larvae to move through bandages: pigs' feet, in a state of decomposition imitating purulent wounds, were placed in plastic boxes with two gravid females of *S. africa*. Two legs were covered with cotton bandages and two others were kept uncovered as controls. After four days, the pig's feet and bandages were examined for the presence of larvae. The results demonstrated the ability of *S. africa* larvae to reach decomposed tissue wrapped in elastic or cotton bandages [61].

The simplest and most effective way to prevent myiasis would be to provide screens for windows and other ventilation ducts. This is particularly important where insects can be attracted during the night-time lighting of a room, as is the case in the intensive care unit. It is also necessary to emphasize the heightened awareness of nursing staff when dealing with serious injuries at a time of year that offers optimum temperature for fly reproduction [58].

Flies are attracted to the genital area for oviposition by odors caused by poor hygiene and coexisting genital infections. It is generally found in people with low levels of education, children and the elderly. Localization in the genital area is generally associated with promiscuous sexual behavior in individuals with multiple sexual partners. Eggs or larvae may be deposited when the patient remains undressed or poorly clothed. This condition can sometimes be observed in tourists visiting exotic destinations in tropical regions such as Central and South America, as well as Africa and Asia. [62].

Human scrotal myiasis was reported in South America due to vinegar fly infestation in a tourist returning from a forested area [63].

Fly larvae can invade the rectum or anus and complete their development inside, in the host's rectum. The most common causes are neglected anal fissure wounds, infectious colitis, polyps and inflammatory bowel disease. Among the flies associated with this phenomenon are *E. tenax* [L.] [Syrphidae] , *F. scalaris* [Fabricius] [Fanniidae], *M. stabulans* [Fallen] [Muscidae] and *Fannia canicularis* [L.] [Fanniidae] [43].

We also cite a case reported by Zardi et al of myiasis of a recto-cutaneous fistula due to *Sarcophaga sp* in a patient suffering from bone metastases in Italy [64].

CONCLUSIONS

Myiasis is defined as "the infestation of living humans and vertebrate animals by dipteran larvae which, for at least a certain period of time, feed on the host's dead or living tissue, liquid body substances or ingested food".

Myiasis has a worldwide distribution and has been reported in many countries, particularly in tropical and subtropical regions, but is extremely rare in the northern hemisphere. In Tunisia, too, it remains a condition rarely encountered and little known by doctors, which makes diagnosis a little difficult. So, with the increase in the number of travellers and, consequently, the rise in imported cases, we'll be faced with this pathology more and more.

The aim of our work was to describe their epidemiological, clinical, evolutionary and therapeutic characteristics.

This was a retrospective, descriptive study involving four cases of myiasis diagnosed at the parasitology-mycology laboratory of the main military training hospital in Tunis.

In our first observation, we report the case of a 38-year-old female patient, a worker at Djerba airport, on corticosteroid and immunosuppressive therapy. The patient presented with clear rhinorrhea, with whitish worms found when blowing her nose. The ENT examination showed only an appearance consistent with congestive rhinitis, and the laboratory work-up was without abnormalities. Macroscopic and microscopic examination of the two larvae identified them as *Oestrus ovis* larvae. The patient was treated with saline nasal lavage several times a day, and progressed well. As for our second observation, it concerned a 50-year-old female patient, a worker at Tunis airport with no notable pathological history. She presented with a flu-like syndrome that had been evolving for 10 days, with polyarthralgia, cough and purulent sputum with whitish worms. ENT examination revealed pharyngitis, and biology and chest X-ray were without abnormality. Parasitological examination identified *Oestrus ovis* larvae. The patient was put on antiseptic mouthwash and saline solution for nasal lavage, with a good evolution. Our third case involved a 60-year-old multitargeted patient treated for a diabetic foot wound in which a whitish worm was found during hyperbaric oxygen therapy. Biology revealed no hypereosinophilia or inflammatory syndrome. A *Lucilia sericata* larva was identified in the parasitology department. The larvae were removed and the wound cleaned with chlorhexidine. The final case involved a 31-year-old patient with no previous history of the disease, who had been involved in a road traffic accident. He was intubated and admitted to the intensive care unit. His evolution was marked by the appearance of a fever with a biological inflammatory syndrome. Several whitish worms were found in his private parts. Parasitological examination identified *Musca Domestica* larvae. The intimate areas were shaved with a conventional toilet and antiseptic disinfection. The patient died on the fourth day after worsening septic shock and multiple visceral failure.

Our study focused on cases of rare myiasis of different types: nasal, wound and nosocomial anal. There were also other cases of myiasis published in Tunisia, notably conjunctival and furuncular. Even when the diagnosis is obvious, some doctors may fail to diagnose it, forcing the patient to take unnecessary treatments such as antibiotics, thus contributing to the increase in antibiotic resistance.

We therefore propose a number of measures:

➔ Promote university and post-graduate training courses on myiasis, particularly in the context of travel medicine.

➔ A pre-travel medical consultation is necessary to advise the traveler on what to avoid and what measures to take to prevent these parasites:

- Encourage travelers in endemic zones to use an iron before wearing clothes left outside.

- Wear long clothing and use mosquito nets.

➔ Curative and preventive treatment of herds with ivermectin [200 µg/kg] appears to be effective in reducing larval infestation. This treatment could reduce the frequency of human estrosis, by at least reducing the risk of contamination from cattle.

➔ Any traveller suspected of having imported myiasis should be systematically and thoroughly questioned, specifying the country of destination, the duration of the trip, the reason for it and the activities undertaken, as well as undergoing a meticulous physical examination. This is the only way to be able to order the necessary additional tests, or even make a diagnosis without carrying out any investigations.

➔ The simplest and most effective way to prevent nosocomial myiasis is to provide screens for windows and other ventilation ducts.

→ It is also necessary to insist on heightened awareness on the part of nursing staff when dealing with serious wounds in a season that offers optimal temperatures for fly reproduction. Wound sites must be inspected and cleaned regularly, and covered with a dressing, to prevent the onset of myiasis.

→ Further studies are needed to better understand the extent of this parasitosis and its real incidence, especially as some may have been treated but not published, despite their rarity.

REFERENCES

1. Zumpt F. Myiasis in man and animals in the old world. London: Butterworths; 1965.

2. Noutsis C, Millikan LE. Myiasis. Dermatol Clin. 1994 Oct;12(4):729-36.

3. Marcondes CB, Thyssen PJ. Myiasis-causing flies. Infect Immun. 2022 Feb;2:924-34.

4. Lachish T, Marhoom E, Mumcuoglu KY, Tandlich M, Schwartz E. Myiasis in travelers. J Travel Med. 2015 Jul;22(4):232-6.

5. Caumes E, Carriere J, Guermonprez G, Bricaire F, Danis M, Gentilini M. Dermatoses associated with travel to tropical countries: a prospective study of the diagnosis and management of 269 patients presenting to a tropical disease unit. Clin Infect Dis. 1995 Mar;20(3):542-8.

6. Thomas S, Nair P, Hegde K, Kulkarni A. Nasal myiasis with orbital and palatal complications. BMJ Case Rep. 2010 Dec;2010:bcr0820103219.

7 Hakeem ML, Bhattacharyya DN. Exotic human myiasis. Travel Med Infect Dis. 2009 Jul;7(4):198-202.

8. Siwar B, Latifa M, Nawel B, et al. Myiasis of wounds caused by Lucilia sericata: First report in Tunisia and literature review. MOJ Clin Med Case Rep. 2021;11(6).

9. Latifa M, Bousbia C, Aïcha R, Nawel B, Boughariou S, Nsiri R, et al. A case report of nosocomial myiasis caused by Musca domestica and literature review. J Clin Med Img. 2022;2:1-4.

10. Association Française des Enseignants de Parasitologie Médicales ANOFEL. Parasitoses and mycoses of temperate and tropical regions. 5th edition. Paris: Masson; 2017.

11. Agoumi A. Précis de parasitologie médicale [Online]. 2003 [cited 22 Sep 2022]. Disponible sur: http://www.sudoc.abes.fr/cbs/xslt/DB=2.1//SRCH?IKT=12&TRM=100501931&COOKIE=U10178,Klecteurweb,D2.1,E5c7cfd05-26a,I250,B341720009+,SY,QDEF,A%5C9008+1,,J,H2-26,,29,,34,,39,,44,,49-50,,53-78,,80-87,NLECTEUR+PSI,R102.24.198.32,FN

12. Scholl PJ, Colwell DD, Cepeda-Palacios R. Myiasis [Muscoidea, Oestroidea]. In Medical and Veterinary Entomology. Academic Press. 2019: p383-419.

13. Guiguen C, Belaz S, Chabasse D, Beaucournu JC. Apport du laboratoire pour le diagnostic des myiases. Rev Francoph Lab. 2020 May;2020(522):72-80.

14. Francesconi F, Lupi O. Myiasis. Clin Microbiol Rev. 2012 Jan;25(1):79-105.

15 Smillie I, Gubbi KS, Cocks HC. Nasal and ophthalmomyiasis: case report. J Laryngol Otol. 2010 Aug;124(8):934-5.

16 Delhaes L, Bourel B, Pinatel F, Cailliez JC, Gosset D, Camus D, et al. Human nasal myiasis caused by *Oestrus ovis*. Parasite. Dec 2001;8(4):289-96.

17. Oestrus ovis [Online]. 2001 [cited 22 Sep 2022]. Available from: https://www.parasite.org.au/pugh-collection/Oestrus%20ovis%20%2001.jpg_Index.html

18. Tahenni S. Myiasis of the nasal cavity (Oestrosis of sheep) [Online]. 2014 [cited 22 Sep 2022]. Available from: https://www.alliance-elevage.com/informations/article/les-myiases-de-la-cavite-nasale-loestrose-des-ovins

19 Pampiglione S, Giannetto S, Virga A. Persistence of human myiasis by Oestrus ovis L. (diptera: oestridae) among shepherds of the etnean area (Sicily) for over 150 years. Parassitologia. 1997 Dec;39(4):415-8.

20. Sergent E. La thimni, myiase oculo-nasale de l'homme cause par l'oestre du mouton. Arch Inst Pasteur Alger. Dec 1952;30(4):319-61.

21. Pagès R. A case of ocular myiasis in poitou. Bull Soc Ophtalmol Fr. 1971 Jul;71(7):743-4.

22 Kilani M, Kacem HH, Dorchies PH, Franc M. Observations on the annual cycle of Oestrus ovis in Tunisia. Rev Med Vet. Mar 1986;137(6):451-7.

23. Anane S, Ben Hssine L. Human conjunctival myiasis caused by Oestrus ovis in southern Tunisia. Bull Soc Pathol Exot. Dec 2010;103(5):299-304.

24. Zayani A, Chaabouni M, Gouiaa R, Ben Hadj Hamida F, Fki J. Conjunctival myiasis. A propos de 23 cas dans le Sahel tunisien. Arch Inst Pasteur Tunis. Oct 1989;66(3-4):289-92.

25. Díez González L, Poncela Blanco M, Mayo Yáñez M. Rhinosinusal myiasis by oestrus ovis third stage larva. Med Clin. 2020 Dec;155(12):566-7.

26. Mumcuoglu KY, Eliashar R. Nasal myiasis due to Oestrus ovis larvae in Israel. Isr Med Assoc J. 2011 Jun;13(6):379-80.

27. Einer H, Ellegård E. Nasal myiasis by Oestrus ovis second stage larva in an immunocompetent man: case report and literature review. J Laryngol Otol. 2011 Jul;125(7):745-6.

28. Baker MC. Green-bottle fly worm infestation of the ear. Myiasis of the ear caused by Phaenica sericata. Laryngoscope. 1953 Jun;63(6):545-8.

29 Sharma H, Dayal D, Agrawal SP. Nasal myiasis: review of 10 years experience. J Laryngol Otol. 1989 May;103(5):489-91.

30. Taylor HM. Screwworm (Cochliomyia americana) infestation in man. Ann Otol Rhinol Laryngol. 1950 Jun;59(2):531-40.

31. Arora S, Sharma JK, Pippal SK, Sethi Y, Yadav A. Clinical etiology of myiasis in ENT: a reterograde period--interval study. Braz J Otorhinolaryngol. 2009 May;75(3):356-61.

32. Kuruvilla G, Albert RA, Job A, Ranjith VT, Selvakumar P. Pneumocephalus: a rare complication of nasal myiasis. Am J Otolaryngol. 2006 Mar;27(2):133-5.

33. Sayeed A, Ahmed A, Sharma SC, Hasan SA. Ivermectin: a novel method of treatment of nasal and nasopharyngeal myiasis. Indian J Otolaryngol Head Neck Surg. 2019 Nov;71 Suppl 3:2019-24.

34 Dorchies P, Alzieu JP, Cadiergues MC. Comparative curative and preventive efficacies of ivermectin and closantel on Oestrus ovis (linné 1758) in naturally infected sheep. Vet Parasitol. 1997 Oct;72(2):179-84.

35. Lucientes J, Castillo JA, Ferrer LM, Peribáñez MA, Ferrer Dufol M, Gracia Salinas MJ. Efficacy of orally administered invermectin against larval stages of Oestrus ovis in sheep. Vet Parasitol. 1998 Feb;75(2):255-9.

36 Wikipedia. Lucilia sericata [Online]. 2021 [cited 22 Sep 2022]. Available from: https://fr.wikipedia.org/w/index.php?title=Lucilia_sericata&oldid=186651626

37. Hall MJ. Trapping the flies that cause myiasis: their responses to host-stimuli. Ann Trop Med Parasitol. 1995 Aug;89(4):333-57.

38. Kotzé Z, Villet MH, Weldon CW. Effect of temperature on development of the blowfly, Lucilia cuprina (Wiedemann) (diptera: calliphoridae). Int J Legal Med. 2015 Sep;129(5):1155-62.

39. Greenberg B. Two cases of human myiasis caused by Phaenicia sericata (Diptera: calliphoridae) in chicago area hospitals. J Med Entomol. 1984 Sep;21(5):615.

40. Terzi AJE. The larva and fly of a greenbottle (Lucilia sericata). [Online]. 2022 [cited 22 Sep 2022]. Available from: https://wellcomecollection.org/works/z8hfj3zg/images?id=fgujcpqv

41. Joo CY, Kim JB. Nosocomial submandibular infections with dipterous fly larvae. Korean J Parasitol. 2001 Sep;39(3):255-60.

42. Uysal S, Ozturk AM, Tasbakan M, Simsir IY, Unver A, Turgay N, et al. Human myiasis in patients with diabetic foot: 18 cases. Ann Saudi Med. 2018 May;38(3):208-13.

43. Singh A, Singh Z. Incidence of myiasis among humans a review. Parasitol Res. 2015 Sep;114(9):3183-99.

44 Bouet G, Roubaud E. Études sur la faune parasitaire de l'Afrique occidentale française. Paris: Masson; 1914.

45. Graham JP, Price LB, Evans SL, Graczyk TK, Silbergeld EK. Antibiotic resistant enterococci and staphylococci isolated from flies collected near confined poultry feeding operations. Sci Total Environ. 2009 Apr;407(8):2701-10.

46. Ranjbar R, Izadi M, Hafshejani TT, Khamesipour F. Molecular detection and antimicrobial resistance of Klebsiella pneumoniae from house flies (Musca domestica) in kitchens, farms, hospitals and slaughterhouses. J Infect Public Health. 2016 Jul;9(4):499-505.

47. Schaumburg F, Onwugamba FC, Akulenko R, Peters G, Mellmann A, Köck R, et al. A geospatial analysis of flies and the spread of antimicrobial resistant bacteria. Int J Med Microbiol. 2016 Nov;306(7):566-71.

48. Onwugamba FC, Fitzgerald JR, Rochon K, Guardabassi L, Alabi A, Kühne S, et al. The role of 'filth flies' in the spread of antimicrobial resistance. Travel Med Infect Dis. 2018 Mar;22:8-17.

49 Emerson PM, Lindsay SW, Walraven GE, Faal H, Bøgh C, Lowe K, et al. Effect of fly control on trachoma and diarrhea. Lancet. 1999 Apr;353(9162):1401-3.

50. Emerson PM, Bailey RL, Mahdi OS, Walraven GL, Lindsay SW. Transmission ecology of the fly Musca sorbens, a putative vector of trachoma. Trans R Soc Trop Med Hyg. 2000 Jan;94(1):28-32.

51. Ramesh A, Bristow J, Kovats S, Lindsay SW, Haslam D, Schmidt E, et al. The impact of climate on the abundance of Musca sorbens, the vector of trachoma. Parasit Vectors. 2016 Jan;9:48.

52. Sesterhenn AM, Pfützner W, Braulke DM, Wiegand S, Werner JA, Taubert A. Cutaneous manifestation of myiasis in malignant wounds of the head and neck. Eur J Dermatol. 2009 Jan;19(1):64-8.

53. Ergün S, Akinci O, Sirekbasan S, Kocael A. Postoperative wound myiasis caused by Sarcophaga carnaria. Turkiye Parazitol Derg. 2016 Sep;40(3):172-5.

54. Nmorsi OP, Agbozele G, Ukwandu ND. Some aspects of epidemiology of filth flies: Musca domestica, Musca domestica vicina, Drosophilia melanogaster and associated bacteria pathogens in Ekpoma, Nigeria. Vector Borne Zoonotic Dis. 2007 Mar;7(2):107-17.

55. Butler JF, Garcia Maruniak A, Meek F, Maruniak JE. Wild Florida house flies (Musca domestica) as carriers of pathogenic bacteria. Fla Entomol. 2010 Jun;93(2):218-23.

56 Terzi AJE. The larva and fly of a house fly (Musca domestica). Coloured drawing by A.J.E. Terzi [Online]. 2020 [cited 22 Sep 2022]. Available from: https://wellcomecollection.org/works/nngbf2ja

57 Sherman RA, Roselle G, Bills C, Danko LH, Eldridge N. Healthcare-associated myiasis: prevention and intervention. Infect Control Hosp Epidemiol. 2005 Oct;26(10):828-32.

58. Daniel M, Šrámová H, Zálabská E. Lucilia sericata (diptera: calliphoridae) causing hospital-acquired myiasis of a traumatic wound. J Hosp Infect. 1994 Oct;28(2):149-52.

59. Adegboye AO, Yakubu AO. Aural myiasis in a 2-week old neonate - case report. Niger Med Pract. 2007 Oct;52(4):94-6.

60. Dutto M, Bertero M. Traumatic myiasis from sarcophaga (bercaeal cruentata meigen, 1826 (diptera, sarcophagidae) in a hospital environment: reporting of a clinical case following polytrauma. J Prev Med Hyg. 2010 Mar;51(1):50-2.

61. Dutto M, Pellegrino M, Vanin S. Nosocomial myiasis in a patient with diabetes. J Hosp Infect. 2013 Jan;83(1):74-6.

62 Petersen CS, Zachariae C. Acute balanoposthitis caused by infestation with cordylobia anthropophaga. Acta Derm Venereol. 1999 Mar;79(2):170.

63. Massey RL, Rodriguez G. Human scrotal myiasis: botfly infestation. Urol Nurs. 2002 Oct;22(5):315-7.

64. Zardi EM, Iori A, Picardi A, Costantino S, Petrarca V. Myiasis of a perineal fistula. Parassitologia. 2002 Dec;44(3-4):201-2.

APPENDICES

Appendix 1

Key to determining myiasis: a diagnostic approach based on clinical forms [10].

1. Maggot clinging to patient at night in Black Africa: *Auchmeromyia senegalensis*. - Maggot from a pseudofuruncle: go to 2 and 3.

2. In a patient returning from West Africa: *Cordylobia anthropophaga*; the cuticular spines cover the entire body of the maggot, the slits are sinuous and converge towards the knob **(figure 20a)**.

3. In a patient returning from Latin America: *Dermatobia hominis*; the maggot's cuticular spines are rosebud-like, forming one row per segment; the respiratory spiracle slits are rectilinear **(Fig. 20b)**. These spines are absent from the last three terminal segments. -Maggot from the false nasal passages or seen on the conjunctiva of the eye: go to 4.

4. The stigmatic orifices are scattered and ponctiform inside the peritreme: *Œstrus* sp. and *Rhinoestrus*. sp. The bud is inserted in the center of the stigma: *Œstrus ovis* **(figure 20c)**.

-The bud is more or less invaginated at the lateral-internal edge of the stigma: Rhinoestrus spp. **(figure 20d)**. Maggot found in stool; stigmas carried by a long posterior filament "rat-tailed larva": *Eristalis tenax*.

5. Maggots from folds, wounds, ear canal, vagina, etc.: go to 6. sinuous stigmatic slits following each other end to end: *Musca domestica* **(figure 20e)**.

6. straight slits converging towards the peritreme button: go to 7.

7. Button set in peritreme: go to 8 **(figures 20f and 20g)**.

-Button not set in peritreme: go to 9.

8. Presence of a tiny buccal sclerite at the apex of the buccal hook: *Calliphora* spp. **(figure 21)**.

9. Absence of a tiny buccal sclerite at the apex of the buccal hook: *Lucilia* ssp. **(figure 22)**.

10. Interrupted peritreme and poorly sclerotized bud: *Cochliomyia* spp. **(figure 20h)**.

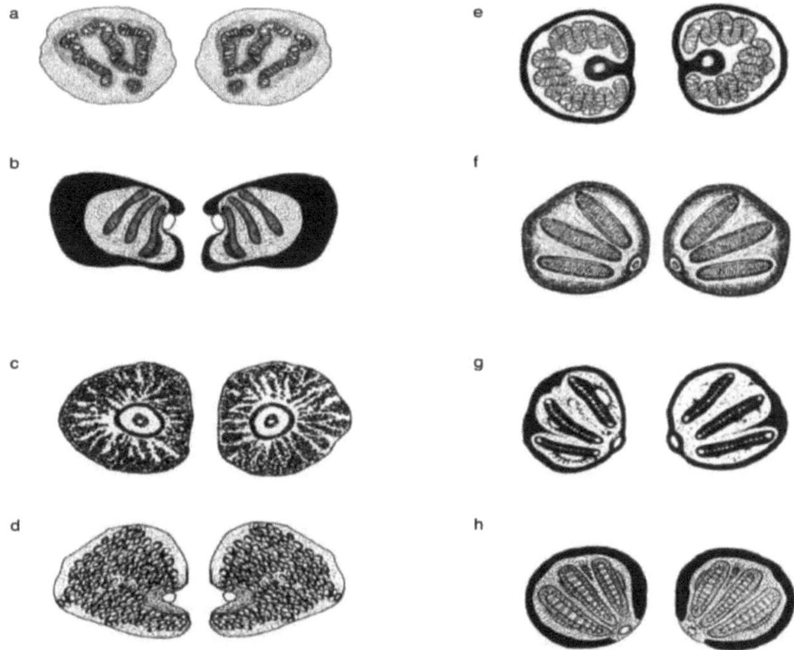

Figure 20. respiratory stigma diagrams

a) *Cordylobia anthropophaga.* b) *Dermatobia hominis.* c) *OEstrus ovis.* d) *Rhinoestrus* spp. e) *Musca domestica.* f) *Calliphora erythrocephala.* g) *Lucilia sericata.* h) *Cochliomyia hominivorax.* [10]

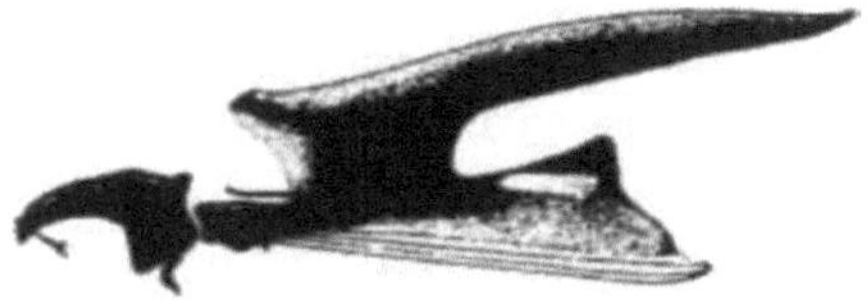

Figure 21. Buccal sclerites of *Calliphora erythrocephala.* [10]

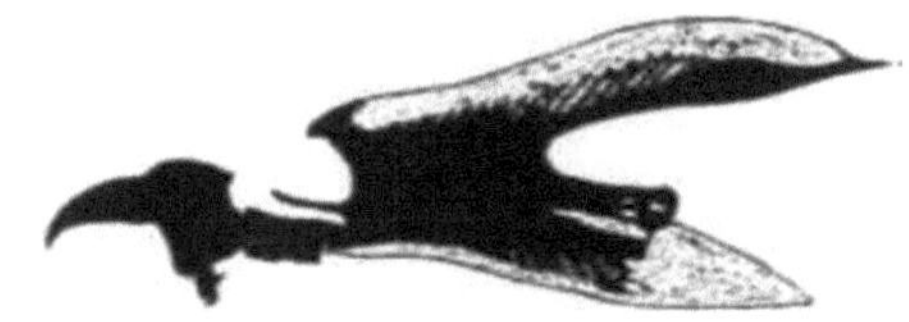

Figure 22. Buccal sclerites of *Lucilia sericata.* [10]

HUMAN MYASIS: A STUDY OF FOUR CASES SEEN IN THE MILITARY HOSPITAL

Summary

Background:

Myiasis is a parasitic infestation of the tissues or body cavities of mammals by dipteran larvae. This ectoparasitosis is of worldwide distribution but represents a disease rarely observed in Tunisia. The aim of our study was to describe the epidemiological, clinical, and biological characteristics of four cases of human myiasis.

Methods:

This was a retrospective descriptive study, collecting four Tunisian cases of myiasis occurring between 2018 and 2022. The diagnosis was made in the laboratory of parasitology-mycology of the military instruction hospital of Tunis by macroscopic and microscopic study according to Zumpt's criteria.

Results:

We reported four Tunisian cases of human myiasis. The average age was 45 years with a sex ratio equal to 1. A history of travel was not reported in our patients. The first two cases represented nasal myiasis due to *Oestrus ovis*. These two patients were employees at the Tunis and Djerba airports. The larvae were extirpated with a good clinical evolution. The third case was myiasis on a diabetic foot wound. The identified larvae were *Lucilia sericata.* The mechanical elimination of the larvae with local care and hyperbaric oxygen therapy allowed healing of the wound. Our last case was a patient who had a nosocomial myiasis of the anus hospitalized in intensive care unit. The species identified was *Musca domestica.* Despite the elimination of larvae with antiseptic disinfection, the outcome was marked by the death of the patient by septic shock and multiple visceral failures.

Conclusion:

Despite the rarity of cases in Tunisia, the diagnosis should not escape us, especially in patients at risk with or without the notion of travel to tropical or subtropical areas. Raising awareness and training healthcare personnel is necessary in order to advise travelers, diagnose and treat these ectoparasitosis.

Key-words Myasis, Nasal cavity, Wounds, Rectum, Tunisia

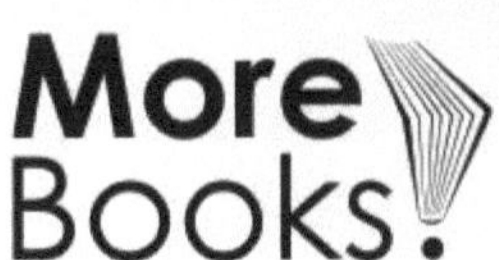

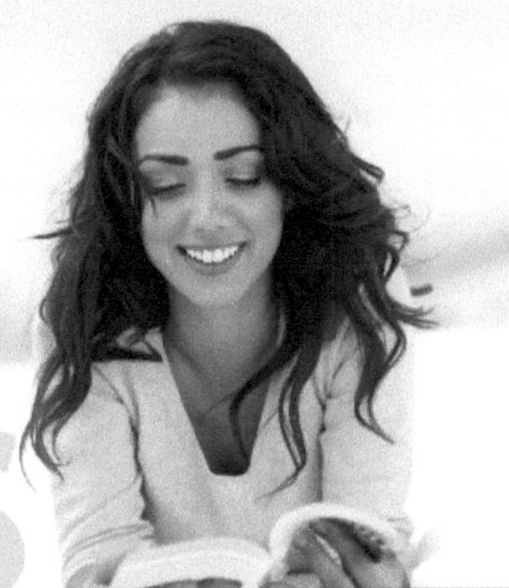

Buy your books fast and straightforward online - at one of world's fastest growing online book stores! Environmentally sound due to Print-on-Demand technologies.

Buy your books online at

www.morebooks.shop

Kaufen Sie Ihre Bücher schnell und unkompliziert online – auf einer der am schnellsten wachsenden Buchhandelsplattformen weltweit! Dank Print-On-Demand umwelt- und ressourcenschonend produziert.

Bücher schneller online kaufen

www.morebooks.shop

info@omniscriptum.com
www.omniscriptum.com

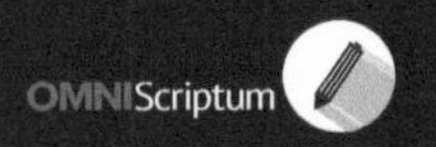

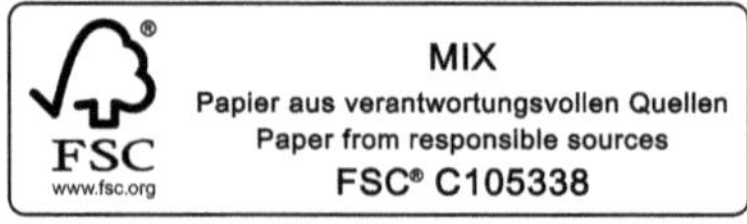

Printed by Books on Demand GmbH, Norderstedt / Germany